Colonel Covid
and the
Army of Antibodies

Written and illustrated by
Hannah Hurley

ISBN 978-1-716-17825-2

A CIP catalogue record for this book is available from the British Library.

All illustrations including front cover design by Hannah Hurley.

Juliette Jones
Editorial Services

Edited and published by Juliette Jones Editorial Services
Juliette.jones@outlook.com

A new nasty germ was about the town.

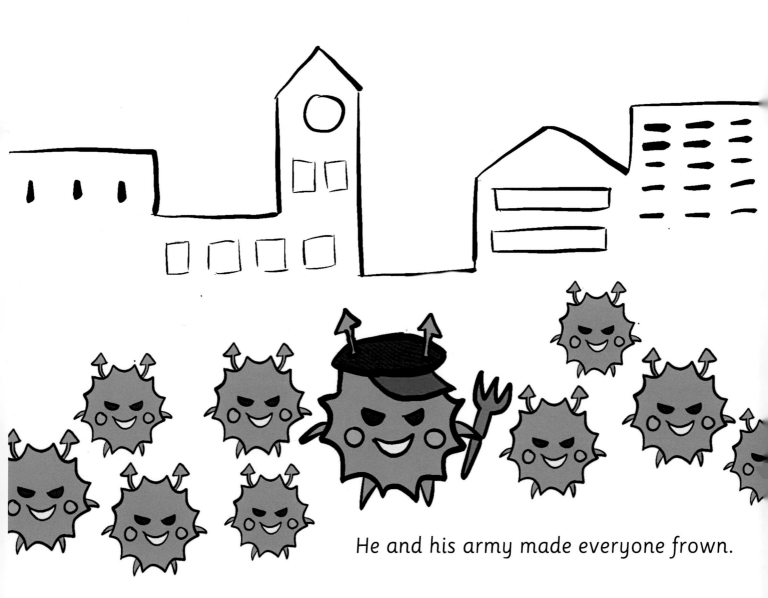

He and his army made everyone frown.

Colonel Covid called loudly and summoned his Army.

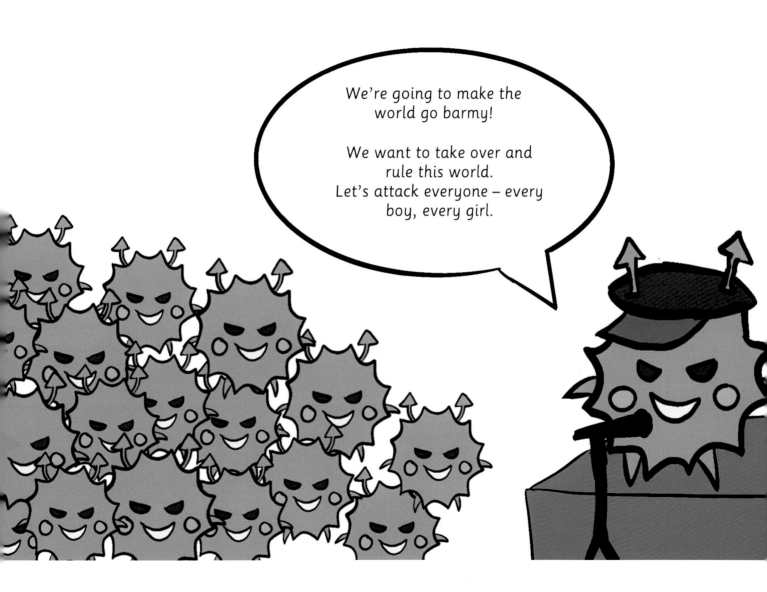

We're going to make the
world go barmy!

We want to take over and
rule this world.
Let's attack everyone – every
boy, every girl.

The troop of germs
made everyone ill.

No medicine could
help them,
not even a pill.

Colonel Covid didn't stop there, his troop travelled afar.

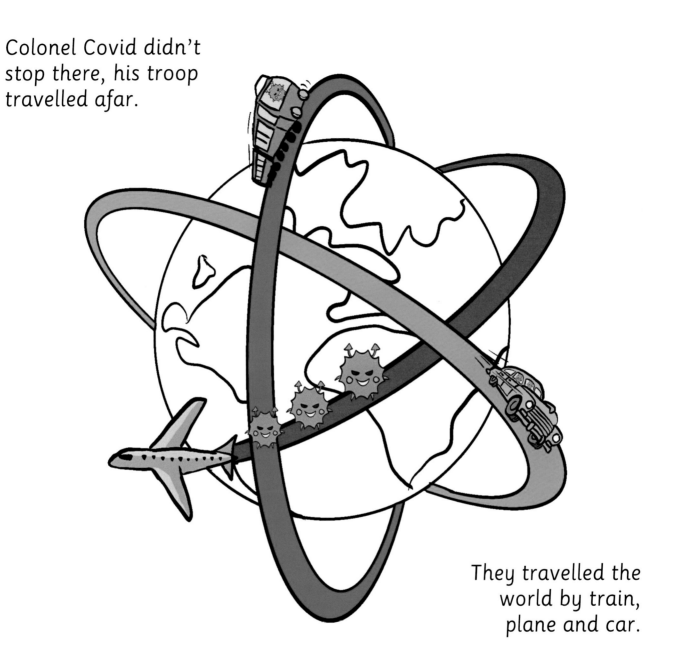

They travelled the world by train, plane and car.

4

They entered into lots of women and men,
making lots of people poorly again and again.

The germ group grew
stronger each and every day.

But ...

... the army in our bodies tried to fight them away.

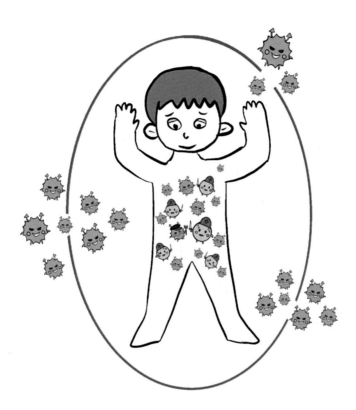

The Army of Antibodies tried their very best.
But the germs were too powerful so they needed to rest.

Colonel Covid had taken over the world and towns.

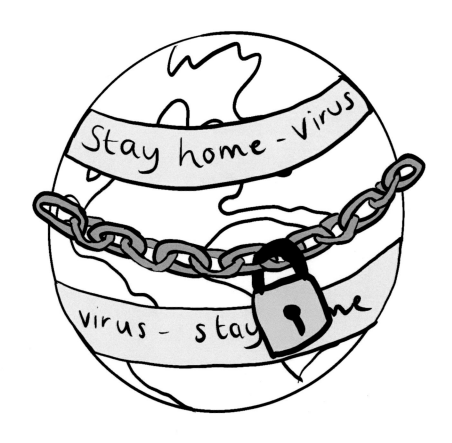

So the people decided it was time to lockdown.

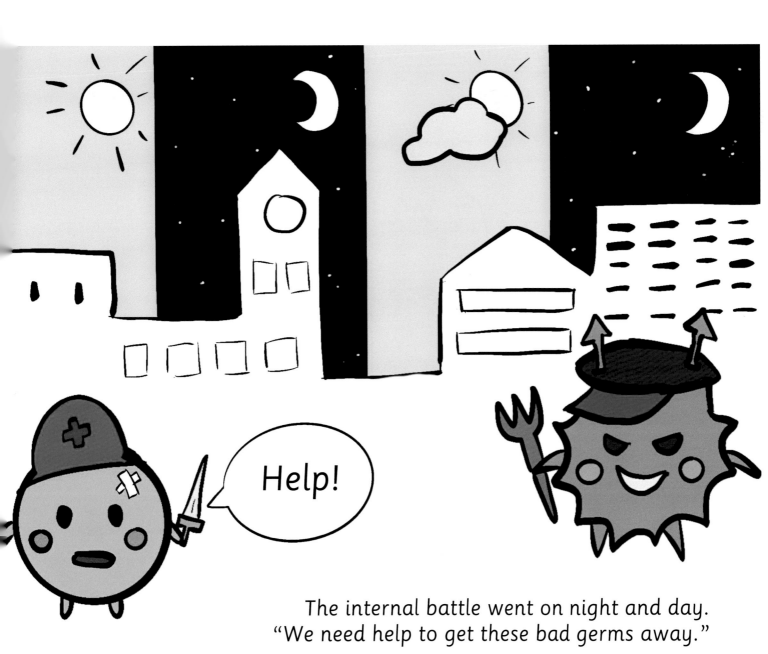

The internal battle went on night and day.
"We need help to get these bad germs away."

Then one day an amazing discovery was made –
A special vaccination that made the germ troop afraid.

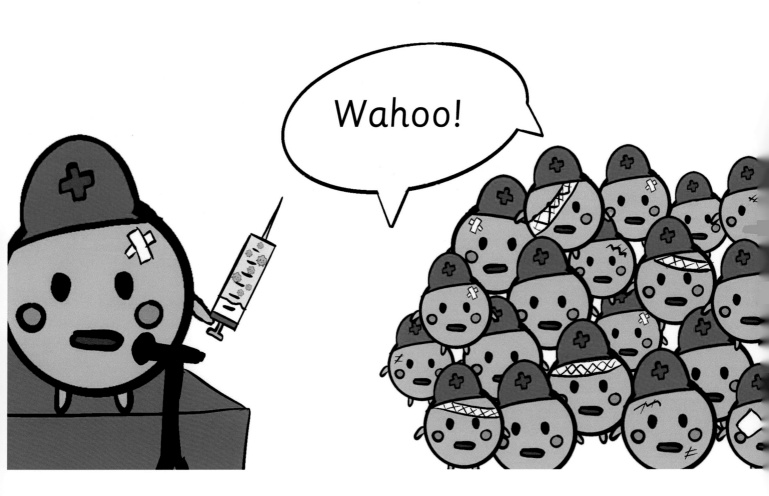

The Army of Antibodies finally had help.
"Wahoo!" they declared, "We've got this!" they yelped.

Slowly but surely the vaccination was given.

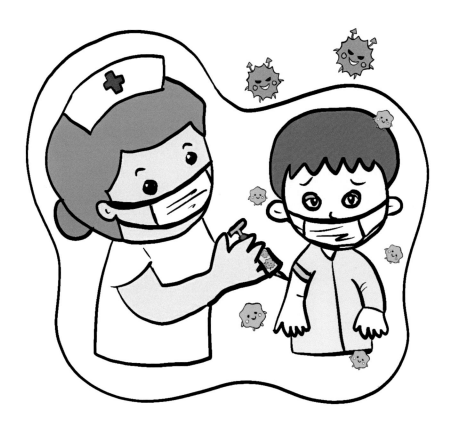

The good guys in our bodies had the stronger position.

The Army of Antibodies grew, grew and grew.
Colonel Covid declared, "We are finally through."

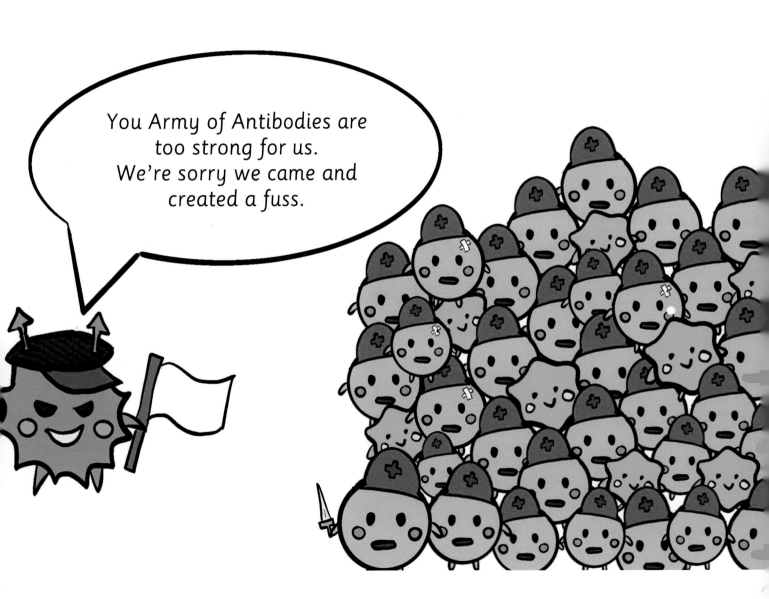

The germ troop had finally given into defeat.
They packed up their things and began to retreat.

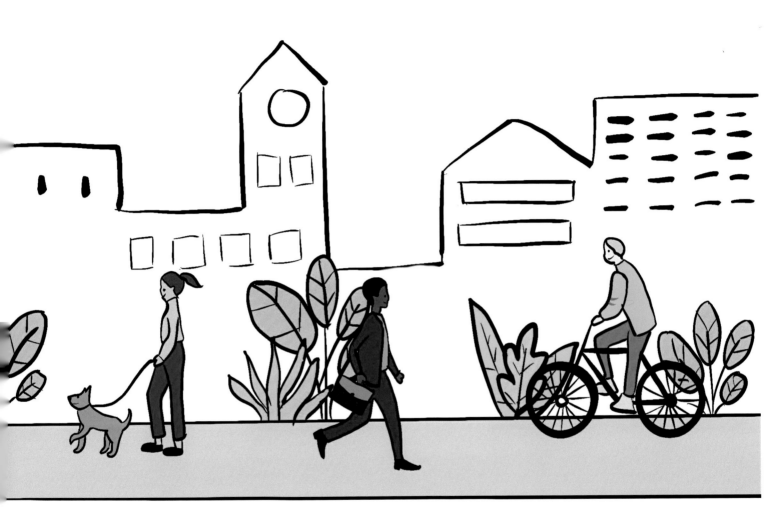

The world returned to normal with each passing day ...

Give a cheer for the Army of Antibodies ...

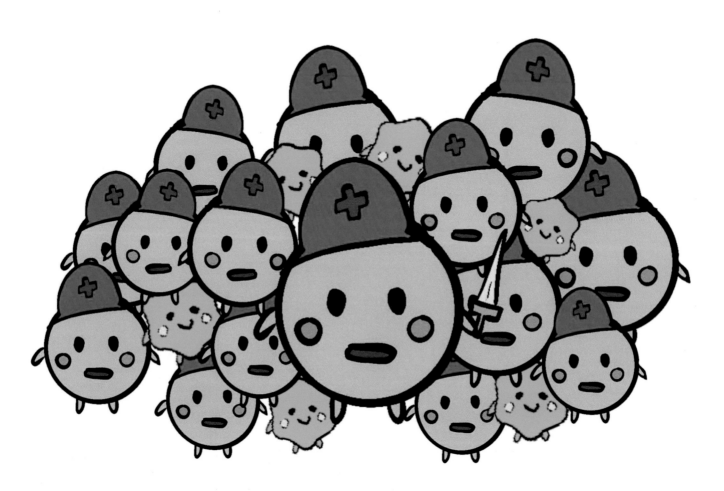

Hip! Hip! Hooray!